FROM MANAGING TO CONQUERING VULVAR CANCER

Expert Guide To Understanding Vulvar Cancer, Unveiling Causes, Recognizing Symptoms, and Embracing Effective Treatments for a Journey to Healthy Living

DR. DASHIELL DANIEL

"Vulvar Cancer," an important resource in the field of oncology, provides a thorough examination of the many facets of vulvar malignancies.

The painstakingly prepared book is an indispensable resource for healthcare professionals, researchers, and individuals seeking a comprehensive grasp of vulvar cancer. The first portion digs into the book's goal, presenting a clear justification for its existence.

It emphasizes the crucial need for enhanced vulvar cancer awareness, early detection, and appropriate treatment—a disease that is sometimes eclipsed by other gynecological cancers.

Chapter 1 establishes the framework for understanding vulvar cancer by describing the vulva's complicated anatomy and categorizing many kinds, including squamous cell carcinoma, melanoma, adenocarcinoma, and unusual variants. This chapter lays the stage for comprehending the signs and symptoms described in Chapter 1.3 by unraveling the complexities of causal causes and risk aspects, underlining the book's commitment to revealing the complexities of vulvar cancer.

The second chapter navigates the diagnostic environment, arguing for screening, early detection, and a thorough analysis of diagnostic techniques like as biopsy, imaging scans, and lymph node appraisal. The disease's stage becomes critical in designing subsequent treatment techniques, easily moving into the section on treatment options that follow. Chapter 3 precisely delineates surgical methods, radiation therapy, chemotherapy, immunotherapy, targeted therapy, and new medicines, ensuring a detailed comprehension of the vulvar cancer therapeutic arsenal.

In Chapter 4, the discussion moves beyond treatment and into the management of treatment-related adverse effects. Recognizing the short- and long-term consequences, the chapter offers insights into pain treatment, tiredness management, and dealing with psychological effects—a comprehensive approach to patient care.

The fifth chapter reveals the process of living with vulvar cancer by providing coping methods, lifestyle changes, and integrative therapies.

The emphasis on emotional support, support groups, counseling, diet, exercise, and integrative therapies demonstrates the book's dedication to a comprehensive approach to patient well-being.

In Chapter 6, survival and follow-up care take center stage, emphasizing the need for recurrence monitoring, survivorship strategies, and physical and emotional well-being issues. Chapter 7 emphasizes the importance of prevention through HPV vaccination, regular check-ups, and public awareness campaigns. Finally, Chapter 8 dives into the frontier of research, revealing ongoing studies, anticipated breakthroughs, and the importance of clinical trials in furthering vulvar cancer understanding and treatment.

Finally, "Vulvar Cancer" goes beyond the bounds of medical literature, providing a nuanced and empathetic analysis of a difficult disease. Its importance stems not just from its academic rigor, but also from its ability to change the face of vulvar cancer management and patient care.

Introduction

Vulvar carcinoma is an uncommon but serious disease that affects the external female genitalia. This book attempts to thoroughly investigate the numerous aspects of overcoming vulvar cancer, providing a detailed explanation of the disease, its epidemiology, risk factors, diagnostics, treatment choices, and the significance of early identification. This book strives to contribute to the information base that can strengthen healthcare professionals, patients, and their families in the fight against vulvar cancer by diving into these topics.

The Book's Purpose

The major goal of this book is to serve as a comprehensive resource that consolidates current vulvar cancer knowledge. The book seeks to provide healthcare professionals with the tools they need for appropriate diagnosis, treatment, and patient care by providing an in-depth analysis of the condition, its origin, and management options. Furthermore, it aims to improve public awareness about vulvar cancer, promoting a greater knowledge of the importance of preventive measures, early detection, and treatment options.

Vulvar Cancer Overview

Vulvar cancer is a type of cancer that begins in the external female genitalia, such as the labia, clitoris, and perineum. It has several histological subgroups, the most common of which is squamous cell carcinoma. Other subtypes, such as melanoma and adenocarcinoma, are less prevalent but present unique diagnostic and therapeutic issues.

Understanding the anatomy and histology of the vulva is critical for healthcare workers caring for vulvar cancer patients. Furthermore, investigating risk factors such as human papillomavirus (HPV) infection, immunosuppression, and chronic inflammatory diseases sheds light on the underlying mechanisms of vulvar carcinogenesis.

Early Detection And Treatment Are Critical

The importance of early identification in the successful management of vulvar cancer cannot be overstated. Given the anatomical position and the possibility of metastasis, a delayed diagnosis can have a major impact on treatment outcomes. This section delves into the numerous early detection approaches, such as clinical examination, colposcopy, and biopsy.

The importance of screening programs, particularly for high-risk populations, in detecting precancerous lesions and initiating prompt therapies cannot be overstated. Vulvar cancer treatment options include surgery, radiation therapy, and chemotherapy, which are frequently used in tandem. Optimizing results requires tailoring treatment regimens to specific patient features and illness stages. Furthermore, addressing the psychosocial components of vulvar cancer, particularly the impact on sexuality and body image, is critical to providing comprehensive patient care.

The Epidemic Of Vulvar Cancer

Understanding vulvar cancer epidemiology lays the groundwork for public health initiatives and focused therapies. This section investigates the global incidence and prevalence of vulvar cancer, taking into account differences across people and geographical locations. Examining trends in age-specific incidence and detecting disparities based on socioeconomic characteristics and healthcare access reveals possible intervention areas. Furthermore, evaluating the influence of high-risk HPV vaccination on vulvar cancer rates is important in the context of preventive efforts.

This book intends to contribute to the creation of evidence-based policies and initiatives to minimize the burden of vulvar cancer by thoroughly evaluating epidemiological data.

Etiology And Risk Factors

Vulvar cancer is impacted by a wide range of risk and etiological variables, including infectious agents and genetic predisposition. The role of HPV infection, particularly high-risk HPV strains, in the development of vulvar squamous cell carcinoma is discussed in this section. Other factors that contribute to the multifactorial character of vulvar cancer include immunosuppression, chronic inflammatory disorders, and smoking. Susceptibility can also be increased by genetic alterations, especially those linked with inherited diseases such as Lynch syndrome.

A thorough understanding of these variables is essential for risk categorization, early identification, and the creation of focused preventative interventions.

Methods Of Diagnosis

Accurate and prompt diagnosis is critical for effective vulvar cancer management. This section delves into the numerous diagnostic methods, such as clinical examination, colposcopy, imaging examinations, and histological evaluation.

Clinical examination, which allows healthcare practitioners to identify suspicious lesions and assess the level of involvement, remains a cornerstone. Colposcopy allows for a more thorough view of the vulva and aids in focused biopsy. Magnetic resonance imaging (MRI) and positron emission tomography (PET) are imaging techniques that help in staging and treatment planning.

Histopathological analysis not only confirms the diagnosis but also gives critical prognostic information. The combination of various diagnostic modalities ensures a thorough and reliable assessment of vulvar cancer cases.

Treatment Options

Vulvar cancer therapy is interdisciplinary, comprising surgical, radiation, and medical oncology methods. Surgery is still the primary therapeutic option, with options ranging from wide local excision in early-stage illness to radical vulvectomy with lymphadenectomy in late cases. The surgical method chosen is determined by criteria such as tumor size, location, and lymph node involvement. Adjuvant therapies, such as radiation therapy and chemotherapy, are frequently used to improve local control while also addressing systemic disease. This section delves deeply into the numerous surgical procedures, radiation protocols, and chemotherapy regimens used to treat vulvar cancer. Furthermore, the significance of a personalized therapy approach that takes into account specific patient variables and preferences is underlined.

Considerations For Psychosocial And Quality Of Life

Vulvar cancer has a psychosocial impact in addition to the physical components of the disease. Addressing patients' emotional and psychological well-being is critical to holistic cancer care. This section delves into the difficulties that patients may confront, such as body image concerns, sexual dysfunction, and the psychological toll of a cancer diagnosis. Implementing supportive treatment measures such as counseling, rehabilitation, and survival programs is critical in enhancing the overall quality of life for vulvar cancer patients. Furthermore, interdisciplinary teams comprised of psychologists, social workers, and sexual health specialists are vital in providing holistic care.

Finally, overcoming vulvar cancer necessitates a holistic approach that includes prevention, early identification, and tailored treatment options.

This book is intended to be a complete resource for healthcare professionals, researchers, and those affected by vulvar cancer.

The book contributes to the expanding landscape of vulvar cancer research and care by digging into epidemiology, risk factors, diagnostic techniques, treatment modalities, and psychosocial aspects. We can improve outcomes, minimize morbidity, and improve overall well-being for patients confronting the challenges of vulvar cancer by continuing to study the illness at both the molecular and clinical levels.

CHAPTER ONE
VULVAR CANCER
UNDERSTANDING

Understanding vulvar cancer begins with understanding the anatomy of the vulva.

The vulva, or female genitalia's exterior section, is made up of several structures, including the mons pubis, labia majora and minor, clitoris, vestibule, and Bartholin's glands. These components work together to accomplish critical reproduction and sexual pleasure functions. awareness of the complexity of vulvar cancer requires a thorough awareness of the vulva's unique structure, as many types of cells and tissues within this region may be affected by malignancies.

Vulvar Cancer Types

Squamous Cell Carcinoma, the most common type of vulvar cancer, develops from the vulva's squamous epithelial cells.

These tumors frequently grow gradually and are linked to precancerous lesions.

Melanoma, another serious kind, develops from pigment-producing cells known as melanocytes. Despite their rarity, melanomas are infamous for their aggressiveness. Adenocarcinoma, a subtype derived from glandular cells, is uncommon but presents unique diagnostic and therapy obstacles. There are also additional rare forms of vulvar malignancies, such as sarcomas and basal cell carcinomas, that require specialist techniques for effective care.

Factors Of Risk And Causes

Investigating the genesis of vulvar cancer entails investigating multiple elements that contribute to its development. Persistent infection with high-risk strains of human papillomavirus (HPV) emerges as a main cause of squamous cell carcinoma, in particular. The interaction of genetic predisposition and environmental circumstances is critical, and certain inherited disorders may increase susceptibility.

Immunocompromised people, such as those with HIV/AIDS, are at a higher risk. Furthermore, smoking, chronic inflammatory disorders, and lichen sclerosis are linked to an elevated risk of vulvar cancer development. A thorough investigation of these causes and risk factors is essential for developing effective preventative and intervention measures.

<u>Symptoms and Signs</u>

Vulvar cancer symptoms show in a variety of ways, often leading to a delayed diagnosis due to patients' unwillingness to address intimate health concerns. Itching, soreness, or tenderness in the vulvar region that persists may signal an underlying problem. Changes in skin color or thickness, the existence of lumps or ulcers, and unusual bleeding are all red signs that should be addressed by a doctor. Furthermore, difficulty urinating or defecating, as well as swollen lymph nodes in the groin, are signs of severe stages. Healthcare practitioners must have a complete grasp of these signs and symptoms to conduct thorough assessments and ensure timely diagnosis and action.

Diagnostic Methodologies

A comprehensive strategy including clinical evaluation, imaging investigations, and pathological testing is used to diagnose vulvar cancer. A thorough examination of the vulva, palpation of inguinal lymph nodes, and assessment of neighboring structures are all part of a comprehensive physical examination.

A biopsy, which is essential in confirming cancer, involves extracting tissue samples for histological investigation. Magnetic resonance imaging (MRI) and computed tomography (CT) scans can help determine the degree of cancer spread. Furthermore, positron emission tomography (PET) scans may be used to evaluate metabolic activity and assist in therapy planning.

The combination of various diagnostic technologies results in a more precise understanding of the disease, allowing healthcare practitioners to modify treatment plans accordingly.

Prognosis And Staging

Staging is critical in evaluating the degree of vulvar cancer and in guiding treatment recommendations. The International Federation of Gynaecology and Obstetrics (FIGO) categorization system is widely utilized, with characteristics such as tumor size, involvement of surrounding structures, and the occurrence of lymph node metastases taken into account.

Vulvar cancer prognosis is impacted by several factors, including the stage of diagnosis, histological subtype, and patient-specific features.

Early-stage vulvar tumors frequently have a better prognosis, with high cure rates achievable by surgical surgery.

Advanced stages involving lymph nodes or distant metastasis, on the other hand, present considerable hurdles, needing multimodal methods such as surgery, radiation therapy, and chemotherapy.

Surgical Procedures

Surgery is still used to treat vulvar cancer, with the amount dictated by the tumor's stage and location. Wide local excision or vulvectomy may be sufficient for early-stage tumors limited to the vulva. Lymph node dissection is used to remove diseased lymph nodes when they are implicated. Surgical advancements, such as sentinel lymph node mapping, attempt to reduce the extent of surgery while assuring optimal oncological results. To improve postoperative functional and cosmetic outcomes, reconstructive surgery may be considered. However, the surgical method is chosen based on the specific characteristics of the tumor and the patient.

Radiation Treatment

Radiation therapy is critical in the treatment of vulvar cancer, especially when surgery alone is insufficient or when cancers infiltrate regional lymph nodes. External beam radiation directs targeted radiation to the afflicted area, destroying cancer cells while sparing healthy tissue.

Another method used to improve local control is brachytherapy, which involves inserting radioactive sources directly into or around the tumor. Radiation therapy must be integrated into the treatment plan through a multidisciplinary approach involving close coordination between radiation oncologists, surgeons, and medical oncologists.

Targeted Therapies And Chemotherapy

Chemotherapy is used to treat vulvar cancer as a main treatment option for advanced or metastatic disease, or as adjuvant therapy after surgery or radiation.

Platinum-based chemotherapy regimens are routinely used to target fast-proliferating cancer cells. The type of chemotherapy used is determined by the features of the tumor as well as the patient's overall condition. Immune checkpoint inhibitors and other targeted medicines are showing promise in the treatment of vulvar cancer. These medicines, which aim to improve the body's immune response to cancer cells, constitute a paradigm shift in cancer treatment. Ongoing research is looking into novel targeted medicines to improve treatment techniques and outcomes.

Survivorship And Multidisciplinary Care

Vulvar cancer treatment requires a multidisciplinary strategy that includes gynecologic oncologists, radiation oncologists, medical oncologists, pathologists, and other healthcare experts. Collaboration among these professionals ensures a thorough examination of the disease, educated treatment recommendations, and the best possible patient care. Furthermore, supportive treatment, such as psychosocial support, symptom management, and rehabilitation services, is critical to meeting the holistic requirements of people diagnosed with vulvar cancer. Survivorship care focuses on the prevention of recurrence, the management of treatment-related adverse effects, and the promotion of overall well-being. Integrating survivorship care plans allows for long-term follow-up and helps survivors negotiate life after vulvar cancer.

To defeat vulvar cancer, a thorough grasp of its anatomy, kinds, causes, and risk factors is required. The foundation for good management is timely detection by knowledge of signs and symptoms, combined with reliable diagnostic procedures. The combination of surgical treatments, radiation therapy, and chemotherapy, as well as new targeted therapeutics, represents the changing landscape of vulvar cancer treatment. A multidisciplinary, holistic approach offers tailored care and addresses the unique needs of individuals diagnosed with this difficult condition. Research advances and current clinical trials continue to impact the future of vulvar cancer management, providing promise for better results and a higher quality of life for those affected.

CHAPITRE TWO
DETECTING VULVAR CANCER

Vulvar cancer is an uncommon but deadly gynecological disease that mostly affects women's external genitalia. The diagnosis of vulvar cancer is an important step in the disease's therapy, and it requires a comprehensive approach that includes screening, diagnostic tests, and staging techniques. Early diagnosis is critical for enhancing treatment results and overall patient prognosis.

Early Detection And Screening

Vulvar cancer screening is not as standardized as it is for other cancers, owing to the disease's rarity and a lack of proven screening techniques.

Early detection, however, remains critical, and healthcare practitioners should be cautious in recognizing risk factors and symptoms during routine gynecological examinations.

Women who have chronic itching, pain, or atypical lesions on the vulva should be assessed as soon as possible, and a high index of suspicion is essential for early detection.

Diagnostic Exams

A biopsy is the most important step in diagnosing vulvar cancer. It entails taking a tiny tissue sample from the worrisome lesion on the vulva.

This sample is then analysed under a microscope to determine the presence of cancer cells, the type of malignancy, and the level of invasion. Following treatment decisions are guided by the biopsy results, which provide critical information about the tumor's characteristics and aggressiveness.

Imaging techniques, including as magnetic resonance imaging (MRI) and computed tomography (CT) scans, are used to determine the extent of the disease and probable metastases. These imaging methods aid in examining the tumor's size and location, assessing its infiltration into surrounding structures, and detecting regional or distant spread. Imaging investigations can help with treatment planning and assessing the overall stage of vulvar cancer.

Lymph Node Evaluation: Because vulvar cancer frequently spreads to regional lymph nodes, assessing the condition of these nodes is crucial for proper staging and therapy decisions.

Sentinel lymph node biopsy is a standard approach for determining lymph node involvement.

The first lymph node(s) to which cancer is expected to spread from the main tumor is identified and removed during this surgery.

Lymph node examination helps to determine the degree of the disease and to plan appropriate treatment measures, such as lymph node dissection if necessary.

Stages Of The Disease

Staging is an important step in the diagnostic process since it determines the extent of the cancer and guides therapy recommendations.

For vulvar cancer, the International Federation of Gynaecology and Obstetrics (FIGO) staging method is often utilized. It takes into account the initial tumor's size and location, lymph node involvement, and the occurrence of distant metastases. Staging assists in categorizing patients into distinct prognosis categories, influencing treatment techniques such as surgery, radiation therapy, and chemotherapy.

Accurate staging is critical for adapting treatment strategies to individual illness characteristics, optimizing therapeutic efficacy, and eliminating needless procedures.

Furthermore, staging helps anticipate the patient's prognosis, allowing healthcare practitioners to give patients and their families accurate expectations about the course of the disease and probable consequences.

vulvar cancer detection requires a multifaceted approach that includes screening, diagnostic tests, and staging methods.

Early diagnosis is critical for enhancing treatment outcomes, particularly by vigilant clinical examination and prompt biopsy. Comprehensive staging ensures that treatment approaches are targeted to the specific characteristics of the disease, increasing the odds of effective management and improving the overall quality of care for vulvar cancer patients.

CHAPTER THREE
TREATMENT OPTIONS

Vulvar carcinoma is an uncommon but serious disease that affects the external female genitalia. To enhance patient results, vulvar cancer care requires a multidisciplinary strategy that incorporates several treatment methods.

Surgery, radiation therapy, chemotherapy, immunotherapy, targeted therapy, and emerging/experimental treatments are among the principal therapeutic options.

Surgery is critical in the treatment of vulvar cancer. Vulvectomy, or surgical removal of part or all of the vulva, is a common treatment for this cancer.

The scope of the vulvectomy is determined by the tumor's size and location. For mild lesions, partial vulvectomy may be sufficient, but radical vulvectomy requires the removal of the entire vulva, often necessitating reconstruction.

Lymph node dissection is usually performed in conjunction with other procedures to determine the amount of disease dissemination and guide future treatment decisions. The goal of this surgical procedure is to accomplish optimal tumor excision while retaining functionality and delivering an acceptable cosmetic outcome.

Another important component in the treatment of vulvar cancer is radiation therapy. External beam radiation and brachytherapy are two prominent methods for targeting the problem area.

Radiation therapy can be used as a stand-alone treatment or in conjunction with surgery, especially in advanced instances or when surgical intervention has considerable morbidity concerns. Radiation therapy is critical for eradicating residual disease, reducing the chance of local recurrence, and maintaining organ function.

Chemotherapy is frequently used in the treatment of vulvar cancer, either as adjuvant therapy after surgery or as a neoadjuvant method to decrease tumors before surgery.

Platinum-based medicines, taxanes, or antimetabolites may be employed as chemotherapeutic agents. Chemotherapy attempts to eradicate cancer cells throughout the body and lower the likelihood of distant metastasis, hence improving total treatment efficacy.

Immunotherapy has emerged as a viable treatment option for a variety of malignancies, including vulvar carcinoma. Immunotherapeutic medicines, such as immune checkpoint inhibitors, function by boosting the immune system of the patient to recognize and fight cancer cells.

This method has promise for patients with vulvar cancer, particularly those with advanced or recurring illnesses, where conventional treatments may be ineffective.

Targeted therapy is a precision medicine method in which specific molecules implicated in cancer growth are targeted.

Targeted therapy for vulvar cancer may target genetic alterations or overexpressed proteins. These medicines aim to interrupt specific cancer-growth pathways, providing a more personalized and less hazardous alternative to standard treatments. This research is ongoing, with potential advances in discovering novel intervention targets.

In the field of emerging and experimental treatments, ongoing research is examining novel methods for vulvar cancer treatment. Clinical trials may look into new medications, combination therapies, or treatment procedures to improve outcomes and reduce side effects.

Before becoming popular alternatives, these experimental medicines are often subjected to a rigorous evaluation procedure to assure their safety and efficacy.

Finally, vulvar cancer treatment is diverse, encompassing surgery, radiation therapy, chemotherapy, immunotherapy, targeted therapy, and experimental medicines.

Treatment options are determined by criteria like as disease stage, tumor features, and patient-specific considerations. Advances in each of these treatment modalities contribute to the changing landscape of vulvar cancer treatment, providing hope for improved survival and quality of life for those affected.

CHAPTER FOUR
MANAGING TREATMENT SIDE EFFECTS

To defeat vulvar cancer, a comprehensive approach is required that goes beyond the primary treatment modalities and includes the management of both short-term and long-term side effects. Addressing these issues is critical to improving the overall quality of life for people undergoing treatment. This discussion will go over how to manage short-term side effects like pain, fatigue, and nausea/vomiting, followed by an in-depth look at long-term side effects like lymphedema, sexual dysfunction, and the psychological impact of vulvar cancer treatment.

Short-term side effects are common in the treatment of vulvar cancer and can have a significant impact on patients' well-being. Pain is a common concern, and managing it is critical to ensuring patient comfort. To alleviate pain, a variety of strategies, including pharmacological interventions and non-pharmacological approaches such as physical therapy and relaxation techniques, are used.

The multidisciplinary nature of cancer care allows for a personalized approach to pain management that takes into account the needs and preferences of the individual patient.

Fatigue is another common short-term side effect experienced by people undergoing vulvar cancer treatment. Cancer-related fatigue has a multifactorial etiology that includes the disease itself, treatment modalities, and psychological factors. Exercise programs, nutritional support, and psychosocial interventions can all help to alleviate fatigue and increase overall energy levels. Healthcare providers must work closely with patients to tailor interventions that address the specific causes of fatigue in each case.

Patients may also experience nausea and vomiting during the short-term phase of vulvar cancer treatment.

Antiemetic medications, dietary changes, and acupuncture are some of the interventions used to treat these symptoms. The unique nature of patient experiences emphasizes the importance of ongoing communication between healthcare providers and patients to adjust interventions as needed and ensure optimal symptom control.

When it comes to long-term side effects, lymphedema is a major concern in the context of vulvar cancer treatment. Surgical procedures and radiation therapy can disrupt the lymphatic system, resulting in lymphatic fluid accumulation and swelling. Manual lymphatic drainage, compression therapy, and patient education are used as management strategies.

These measures are intended not only to reduce existing lymphedema but also to prevent its progression and recurrence.

Sexual dysfunction is a complex and multifaceted long-term side effect that can have a significant impact on the quality of life of vulvar cancer patients. Sexual difficulties can be exacerbated by surgical interventions and the psychological impact of cancer. To address sexual dysfunction, open communication between patients and healthcare providers is required, as well as the inclusion of psychosexual counseling, rehabilitation programs, and, if necessary, medical interventions. To restore and improve sexual well-being, an integrated approach that considers both physical and psychological aspects is required.

Vulvar cancer and its treatment have a psychological impact that extends beyond sexual dysfunction to include broader mental health concerns. Cancer survivors are prone to anxiety, depression, and post-traumatic stress disorder (PTSD). Psychosocial support, counseling, and support groups are critical in addressing these issues. Integrating mental health support into the overall care plan is critical for promoting resilience and coping strategies among vulvar cancer survivors.

conquering vulvar cancer necessitates not only the effective implementation of primary treatment modalities but also a comprehensive approach to managing the wide range of short- and long-term side effects. Each aspect, from pain and fatigue to lymphedema, sexual dysfunction, and psychological impact, necessitates a nuanced and personalized approach.

Multidisciplinary collaboration among healthcare providers, including oncologists, pain specialists, physical therapists, psychologists, and counselors, is critical to achieving optimal outcomes and improving the overall well-being of vulvar cancer patients. Continuous research, education, and patient-centered care can help to refine and advance the management of vulvar cancer side effects, ultimately improving the lives of those who have had or are having treatment for this difficult condition.

CHAPTER FIVE
LIVING WITH VULVAR CANCER

Living with vulvar cancer can be a difficult journey that necessitates the use of various coping strategies to address the disease's emotional, psychological, and physical aspects. In terms of coping strategies, emotional support is critical in assisting individuals in navigating the complexities of vulvar cancer.

A cancer diagnosis has a significant emotional impact, and patients benefit greatly from the support of family, friends, and healthcare professionals. The compassionate guidance of healthcare providers and the empathetic understanding of loved ones contribute to a patient's emotional well-being, fostering resilience in the face of the challenges posed by vulvar cancer.

Individuals suffering from vulvar cancer can also benefit from support groups. These groups provide a forum for patients to share their experiences, exchange coping strategies, and gain insights into dealing with the disease's unique challenges. Participation in support groups not only provides emotional solace but also fosters a sense of community, reducing feelings of isolation that cancer patients frequently experience. Individuals with vulvar cancer can find strength in shared experiences by connecting with others who understand their struggles, empowering them to face the uncertainties of their journey.

Counseling is emerging as an important component of vulvar cancer patients' coping strategies. Professional counseling services provide individuals with a structured and confidential environment in which to express their fears, anxieties, and concerns. Patients can benefit from the assistance of mental health professionals with specialized training in cancer-related issues in developing coping mechanisms, addressing psychological distress, and improving their overall quality of life. Counseling sessions may include a variety of therapeutic approaches, such as cognitive-behavioral therapy, to provide patients with effective tools for dealing with the emotional effects of vulvar cancer.

Lifestyle changes, in conjunction with coping strategies, are important in the overall management of vulvar cancer. Nutrition is critical in supporting cancer patients' overall well-being. Dietary choices can have an impact on treatment outcomes as well as the body's ability to cope with the side effects of cancer therapies.

A well-balanced, nutrient-dense diet helps to maintain strength, manage weight, and promote optimal immune function. Nutritional counseling becomes an important part of the overall care plan, tailoring dietary recommendations to the specific needs and challenges that people with vulvar cancer face.

Exercise is another important component of lifestyle changes that can benefit vulvar cancer patients. Physical activity regularly helps to improve physical functioning, mood, and fatigue. Individualized exercise programs, guided by healthcare professionals, consider the individual's overall health status as well as treatment-related considerations.

Participating in appropriate exercise regimens not only promotes physical well-being but also empowers patients by instilling control over their bodies and health outcomes.

Integrative therapies include a variety of complementary approaches that can be incorporated into the overall care plan for patients with vulvar cancer. These therapies, which may include acupuncture, massage, yoga, and meditation, are intended to address the holistic needs of cancer patients. Integrative therapies can help with treatment-related side effects, pain management, and overall well-being. While these approaches are not intended to be replacements for conventional medical treatments, their inclusion in the treatment plan reflects a patient-centered approach that recognizes the importance of addressing the mind-body connection in the context of vulvar cancer.

To summarize, the multifaceted nature of vulvar cancer necessitates a comprehensive approach to addressing the disease's physical, emotional, and lifestyle dimensions. Coping strategies, such as emotional support, support group participation, and counseling, serve as the foundation for navigating the emotional challenges associated with vulvar cancer. Nutrition, exercise, and integrative therapies all contribute to patients' overall well-being by promoting resilience and empowering individuals to actively participate in their care. By embracing these ideas, healthcare providers can improve the quality of life for people living with vulvar cancer, fostering a patient-centered and holistic approach to cancer care.

CHAPTER SIX
SURVIVAL AND FOLLOW-UP CARE

Survivorship after vulvar cancer treatment entails a comprehensive approach that includes recurrence monitoring, survivorship plans, and considerations for physical health, emotional well-being, and long-term health.

Regular examinations and imaging studies are used to monitor for recurrence, which is an important aspect of post-treatment care. Physicians closely monitor any signs of cancer recurrence, using a combination of clinical assessments, imaging techniques, and biomarker assessments to detect early signs of recurrence. The vigilant monitoring strategy aims to intervene quickly if a recurrence is detected, increasing the likelihood of successful treatment.

Survivorship plans are critical to ensuring the well-being of people who have overcome vulvar cancer. These plans, which are tailored to each patient's specific circumstances, cover a wide range of topics, including physical health, emotional well-being, and long-term health considerations.

To monitor overall health and address any emerging health issues, survivorship plans include regular medical check-ups, gynecologic examinations, and imaging studies. These plans also include advice on lifestyle changes, such as eating a healthy diet and exercising regularly, to promote overall well-being and reduce the risk of potential complications.

Emotional well-being is an important aspect of survivor care. Defeating vulvar cancer can have profound psychological consequences, and survivorship plans frequently include psychosocial support services. Counseling, support groups, or therapy sessions may be used to assist individuals in navigating the emotional challenges that may arise following treatment. Addressing anxiety, depression, and other mental health issues is critical for survivors to develop a positive and resilient mindset.

Long-term health concerns are an important part of survivorship planning. These concerns go beyond the immediate post-treatment period and focus on the long-term effects of cancer and its treatments. Physicians work with survivors to create plans that address potential long-term effects such as infertility, hormonal imbalances, and other health conditions that may emerge years after treatment. Regular health screenings and assessments are used to detect and effectively manage these long-term effects.

Checking For Recurrence

Monitoring for recurrence is a time-consuming process that includes clinical assessments, imaging investigations, and biomarker analysis. Regular gynecologic examinations, during which healthcare experts check the vulvar region for any indicators of abnormalities, are part of clinical evaluations. Imaging investigations such as computed tomography (CT) scans, magnetic resonance imaging (MRI), and positron emission tomography (PET) scans may also be used to see internal structures and identify potential areas of concern.

Biomarker analyses are critical in recurrence monitoring. Increased levels of specific biomarkers in blood tests may indicate the presence or recurrence of cancer. Squamous cell carcinoma antigen (SCC-Ag), a tumor marker specific to vulvar cancer, is frequently examined to provide further information on the disease status.

Using a combination of these monitoring tools allows healthcare practitioners to detect potential recurrences at an early stage, boosting the likelihood of successful intervention and treatment.

The frequency of recurrence monitoring differs depending on individual risk factors, the stage of the initial cancer, and the exact treatment taken. Follow-up meetings with healthcare experts, especially gynecologic oncologists, are organized regularly to ensure that any potential indicators of recurrence are identified and managed as soon as possible. This vigilant monitoring technique gives survivors a sense of security while also allowing for timely intervention if any issues occur.

Survivorship Strategies

Survivorship plans are tailored, all-inclusive solutions developed to meet the different requirements of people who have successfully beaten vulvar cancer. Recognizing the varied nature of survivorship, these plans include physical health, emotional well-being, and long-term health issues. Survivorship plans are created through collaboration between healthcare experts, survivors, and their support networks to build a holistic framework for ongoing care.

Physical Fitness

Physical health survivorship strategies include frequent medical check-ups and gynecologic examinations to monitor overall health and detect any potential concerns.

Gynecologic oncologists play an important role in survivorship treatment, including thorough examinations of the vulvar region and adjacent areas to ensure that no evidence of cancer recurrence or other gynecologic disorders exists. Survivors may also be subjected to imaging studies, such as pelvic ultrasounds or CT scans, to collect thorough information about the pelvic region and identify any abnormalities.

It is critical to incorporate lifestyle changes into survivorship programs to promote overall well-being. Guidance on eating a balanced diet, getting enough exercise, and avoiding tobacco and excessive alcohol usage all contribute to survivors' general health. These lifestyle guidelines are intended to lower the likelihood of comorbidities and strengthen the body's resilience following cancer therapy.

Emotional Wellness

The emotional toll of vulvar cancer is significant, and survivorship plans emphasize the necessity of addressing the psychological components of healing. Psychosocial support services, including counseling and support groups, are frequently included in survivorship plans to help people cope with the emotional issues that can develop after treatment. Mental health specialists work with survivors to help them develop coping methods, manage anxiety or sadness, and cultivate a positive attitude.

Survivorship plans include educational components to help survivors comprehend the emotional aspects of healing. This may entail supplying materials on coping processes, stress management approaches, and ways for maintaining a positive attitude in life.

Giving survivors the knowledge and resources, they need to manage the emotional intricacies of survivorhood is essential for promoting resilience and emotional well-being.

Considerations For Long-Term Health

Survivorship plans look beyond the immediate post-treatment phase to address potential long-term health issues. These concerns stem from the influence of cancer and its therapies on numerous areas of health, such as fertility, hormonal balance, and the chance of acquiring other health problems.

Fertility concerns may arise for certain vulvar cancer survivors, particularly if reproductive organs or systems are damaged after therapy. Before treatment, survivorship plans may include discussions about fertility preservation alternatives, as well as continued monitoring of reproductive health after treatment. Fertility specialists may be consulted to investigate assisted reproduction technologies or other family planning options.

Hormonal imbalances are another factor to consider in survivorship planning, especially if hormonal medications were used as part of the treatment program. Overall health and well-being must monitor hormone levels and rectify any abnormalities. Endocrinologists and gynecologic oncologists may work together to effectively manage the hormonal components of survival.

To detect and manage potential late effects of cancer treatment, survivorship programs include regular health exams and assessments.

Based on individual risk factors and treatment history, these screenings may include bone density scans, cardiovascular exams, and other procedures. Detecting and managing long-term health concerns early on improves the overall health and quality of life of vulvar cancer survivors.

Finally, vulvar cancer survivability and follow-up care necessitate a comprehensive and tailored strategy. Individuals who have overcome vulvar cancer benefit from thorough monitoring for recurrence, and survivorship strategies that include physical health, emotional well-being, and long-term health considerations. The incorporation of medical, emotional, and lifestyle components in survivorship plans aims to assist survivors in leading healthy and satisfying lives after their cancer experience is completed.

CHAPTER SEVEN
PREVENTION AND AWARENESS
Vaccination Against The Human Papillomavirus (HPV)

Vulvar cancer prevention begins with addressing the root cause, and infection with high-risk strains of Human Papillomavirus (HPV) is one of the most significant risk factors for vulvar cancer. Vaccination against HPV has emerged as a critical technique for lowering vulvar cancer incidence. The HPV vaccine primarily targets the strains that cause the vast majority of cervical cancers, but it also offers significant protection against vulvar cancer. This precaution is especially important in children, as the vaccination is most effective when given before viral exposure. Public health initiatives should concentrate on expanding access to the HPV vaccine, stressing its significance not only in preventing cervical cancer but also in lowering the overall burden of HPV-related malignancies, including vulvar cancer.

The HPV vaccine's safety and efficiency have been repeatedly proved in studies, making it a vital tool in the fight against vulvar cancer.

Early Detection And Routine Examinations

Early identification is critical to the successful treatment of vulvar cancer. A thorough prevention strategy must include regular check-ups and screenings. Women should be encouraged to have routine gynecological exams, such as pelvic exams and Pap screenings, to detect precancerous abnormalities in the vulva. The need for self-examination should also be emphasized, as it allows women to become acquainted with their bodies and report any unusual changes to their healthcare practitioners. Early detection not only increases the likelihood of successful therapy, but it can also decrease the need for extensive procedures and improve overall prognosis. Healthcare professionals play an important role in teaching women about the signs and symptoms of vulvar cancer, making them aware of the significance of regular screenings, and encouraging them to take a proactive approach to their reproductive health.

Initiatives To Raise Public Awareness

Effective vulvar cancer prevention necessitates powerful public awareness campaigns that refute misunderstandings and encourage proactive health-seeking behaviors. Public health campaigns should try to promote knowledge about the risk factors for vulvar cancer, with a focus on HPV, smoking, and immunosuppression. Furthermore, educating the public about the necessity of proper genital hygiene and recognizing early warning signals is critical. These campaigns should be tailored to different communities, taking cultural and socioeconomic aspects into account that may influence healthcare-seeking behaviors.

Collaboration among healthcare professionals, advocacy groups, and educational institutions is critical to the success of these public awareness campaigns.

To build a complete and persistent effort in preventing vulvar cancer, public awareness activities should go beyond standard media channels and include community outreach programs, educational seminars, and partnerships with healthcare practitioners.

Finally, the preventative and awareness techniques listed above are essential components of a holistic approach to vulvar cancer treatment. Implementing HPV vaccination programs, combined with early identification through frequent check-ups and aggressive public awareness campaigns, has the potential to drastically reduce the prevalence of vulvar cancer.

These interventions contribute to a complete framework for preventing vulvar cancer and improving overall women's health outcomes by targeting both primary risk factors and promoting a culture of proactive reproductive health.

CHAPTER EIGHT
VULVAR CANCER
RESEARCH AND ADVANCES

Vulvar cancer, an uncommon but deadly gynecological malignancy, has been the subject of intensive research to better understand its etiology, development, and treatment options. Ongoing research on vulvar cancer includes molecular biology, genetics, epidemiology, and immunology. Researchers are looking at the genetic variables that may predispose people to vulvar cancer to find particular mutations or biomarkers that may be used as diagnostic or prognostic signs. Furthermore, research is being conducted to investigate the impact of viral infections, such as human papillomavirus (HPV), in the development of vulvar cancer, to provide light on potential preventive methods.

A better understanding of vulvar cancer's molecular and cellular mechanisms has resulted in promising breakthroughs.

The identification of particular pathways implicated in vulvar carcinogenesis has been made possible by advances in genomics and proteomics, paving the way for tailored therapeutics.

Immunotherapeutic treatments for vulvar cancer that use the body's immune system to target and eliminate cancer cells have shown promise in preclinical and early clinical trials.

These discoveries not only provide novel therapeutic choices but also contribute to personalized medicine by adapting interventions to specific genetic profiles.

Clinical trials are critical in converting research findings into measurable improvements in patient outcomes. Current vulvar cancer clinical trials are examining novel therapy techniques such as targeted treatments, immunotherapies, and combination approaches.

These studies attempt to evaluate the safety and efficacy of new treatments, giving crucial data that will help to shape future standards of care. Furthermore, clinical trials investigate how to improve existing treatments, such as surgery and radiation therapy, while minimizing side effects. Enrolling patients in clinical trials is critical for developing the field and providing patients with access to cutting-edge medicines.

CONCLUSION

In conclusion, vulvar cancer research has made considerable advances in recent years, contributing to a more thorough understanding of the illness and enabling novel therapeutic options. Ongoing research efforts continue to elucidate the complex biochemical and genetic mechanisms that underpin vulvar carcinogenesis, thereby giving prospective targets for therapeutic approaches. Promising advances in genomics and immunotherapy, in particular, provide the potential for more effective and tailored treatments, ushering in an era of customized care for vulvar cancer patients.

As a critical component of translational research, clinical trials bridge the gap between laboratory findings and clinical applications.

These studies seek to enhance the results and quality of life of vulvar cancer patients by evaluating the safety and efficacy of future medicines as well as refining conventional treatment regimens. In the world of clinical trials, collaboration between researchers, doctors, and patients is critical to developing the field and bringing innovative treatments to the forefront of cancer care.

As we look ahead, the interdisciplinary aspect of vulvar cancer research will remain critical. Integrating insights from molecular biology, immunology, and clinical oncology will allow for a more thorough knowledge of vulvar cancer, allowing for the creation of comprehensive and customized treatment methods.

Furthermore, recent efforts in preventive measures, such as HPV vaccination, highlight the significance of a multimodal approach to vulvar cancer treatment and prevention.

In essence, collective progress in vulvar cancer research and clinical treatment demonstrates the scientific community's tenacity in handling challenging oncological challenges.

The knowledge generated from current research, promising breakthroughs, and clinical trials collectively shapes the growing landscape of vulvar cancer management, providing hope for better outcomes and a brighter future for those impacted by this condition.